Distribution, publication, and copying in any form are prohibited and subject to damages.

TEN HYPNOSES

Copying, publishing, and sharing with third parties are only permitted with the written consent of the author. Please observe the notes on copyright and usage.

Distribution, publication, and copying in any form are prohibited and subject to damages.

Copying, publishing, and sharing with third parties are only permitted with the written consent of the author. Please observe the notes on copyright and usage.

Ingo Michael Simon

TEN HYPNOSES

26
Fear of Flying, Aviophobia

Distribution, publication, and copying in any form are prohibited and subject to damages.

© 2024 Ingo Michael Simon
All rights reserved.
Independently published
www.ingosimon.com

Important Notes for Urgent Attention:

The contents of this book are based on the practical experiences of the author with hypnosis applications and psychotherapy in a trance state. Although the author has strived for the utmost care, errors or misunderstandings in the presentation cannot be completely excluded. Therapeutic work with people and the application of hypnosis are solely the responsibility of the hypnotist. It cannot be ruled out that parts of this book may be misunderstood or that the application of a presented procedure may cause an undesirable reaction in the client. The author also assumes no co-responsibility if work with a client is carried out with reference to the statements in this book.

The Author:

Ingo Michael Simon studied psychology and education and is a hypnotherapist with practices in southwestern Germany and Switzerland. With the help of hypnosis-supported psychotherapy, he primarily treats people with persistent psychological conditions. His practice focuses on anxiety disorders, pathological compulsions, and psychosomatic illnesses. His therapeutic offerings mainly include classical and modern hypnosis applications and the dreamland therapy he developed himself.

Copying, publishing, and sharing with third parties are only permitted with the written consent of the author. Please observe the notes on copyright and usage.

Distribution, publication, and copying in any form are prohibited and subject to damages.

INTRODUCTION	6
COPYRIGHT AND USAGE	8
HYPNOSIS 1	10
HYPNOSIS 2	15
HYPNOSIS 3	22
HYPNOSIS 4	28
HYPNOSIS 5	33
HYPNOSIS 6	39
HYPNOSIS 7	44
HYPNOSIS 8	50
HYPNOSIS 9	56
HYPNOSIS 10	61
ALL TITLES IN THE SERIES	66

Copying, publishing, and sharing with third parties are only permitted with the written consent of the author. Please observe the notes on copyright and usage.

Introduction

The series "Ten Hypnoses" is very well known in Germany, Austria, and Switzerland as a collection of texts for therapeutic work and is used by numerous psychotherapeutic practices, doctors, therapists, coaches, and other helping professionals. I am pleased to now be able to offer these texts in other countries as well.

Most therapists have their own methods for inducing and deepening trance as well as for exiting trance. Therefore, I have focused on the main part of the hypnosis. The texts in this book can be integrated as the main part into any hypnosis process. The texts in this collection use various hypnosis techniques. I will not explain these in detail, as I assume that users have the appropriate training. It is also not necessary to understand the exact structure or functioning of the different parts. The texts can simply be read aloud, and they will have their effect.

Decide for yourself which text best suits your client or patient at any given time. You can also combine passages from different texts. It is not about using all ten hypnoses in sequence. It is a selection of possibilities.

I want to emphasize that books cannot replace therapy. Psychotherapy or other therapeutic treatments involve much more. A careful diagnosis is the necessary basis for deciding on the use of methods, including whether hypnosis or one of my texts should be used. Even in this case, preparatory discussions, follow-up discussions during the session, and of course, a therapeutic concept for the sequence of sessions and the content approaches are essential parts of therapy. This cannot and should not be achieved with a collection of texts.

In any case, I wish you much success in your work and I am pleased if my text templates can contribute in a small way.

Ingo Michael Simon

Copyright and Usage

Copying, publishing, and sharing with third parties is prohibited and only permitted with the written consent of the author. Please observe the following copyright and usage guidelines.

This work has been carefully crafted and created to the best of the author's knowledge and personal experience. It comprises text templates and application guidelines for professional hypnosis sessions. The author is a licensed psychotherapist with extensive experience in psychotherapy, coaching, and personal training using hypnotic techniques and methods. Nevertheless, the author and the publisher assume no liability for the accuracy of information, instructions, and advice, nor for any typographical errors. The author and publisher accept no responsibility or liability for the application of these texts and recommendations with clients or patients, nor for any potential consequences or unexpected reactions. It is expressly noted that the application of therapeutic and advisory techniques and formulations lies solely and entirely within the responsibility of the practitioner. This also applies to adherence to the boundaries of legally regulated medical and therapeutic practices. The fact that a book containing action proposals is freely available for sale does not imply that its application with clients or patients is permitted for everyone.

Hypnosis 1

You want to fly on an airplane and feel comfortable doing so... You have this clear goal and you are fully committed to it... preparing yourself mentally to let go of this fear today... to end the fear of flying... because it is your will... because it is your declared will... and nothing is stronger than true willpower... and today you succeed remarkably well in making this will so strong... and making this will to overcome fear the strongest will within you...

It's impressive how well you can focus on making this your most important goal of the day... your most important goal of all... Letting go of fear, that is your goal... Letting go of the fear of flying, that is your goal... your most important goal... and nothing and no one can prevent you from pursuing this goal... nothing and no one can slow you down in letting go of the fear... Today is the day... Today is the end of fear... today is the end of the fear of flying... You have decided... You have the power... You let go of fear... You build courage and strength... You win...

Fear can be a feeling or a thought... often it is a thought that convinces us that we are afraid... or several thoughts... thoughts that we formulate as questions... What if? ... What could happen? ... and so on... Enough of that, because these are not feelings... They are just thoughts, and thoughts can be changed... much faster than real feelings... So let's replace the fearful thought with a strong and confident thought... with a thought of courage... You focus on the thought that tells you... I can and will fly whenever and wherever I want... This is the thought of courage and confidence... the thought of your strength... because this strength is indeed within you... You bring it to the forefront, making it the thought of the day and the guiding principle for the time ahead... I can and will fly whenever and wherever I want... This is your thought... This is your personal thought... I can and will fly whenever and wherever I want... Very good... This thought helps you to actually fly with a sense of safety...

Your body helps you... Your body moves into a state of relaxation... You can already feel the relaxation, sensing that you are calm and composed; it's quite clear now, no matter what you might be thinking about... Calmness remains... and your body always follows your thoughts... The more you think of calmness, the calmer your body becomes... and the more you think your new thought, the stronger your body becomes... and a strong body posture makes you even stronger inside... You think... I can and will fly whenever and wherever I want... and your body becomes tall and strong... because that's exactly how you are inside... tall and strong... truly tall and very strong...

Feelings also follow our thoughts when the thought is good and constructive... and your thought of courage and confidence is indeed a good thought... a truly constructive thought... your thought that you can and will fly is a really good thought... and your thought that you can and will fly is truly a constructive thought... so this feeling of calmness becomes more intense... so the feeling of ease while flying becomes more intense... so the feeling of courage within you grows stronger... so the feeling of confidence and inner strength becomes increasingly stable and greater within you... You are ready... you are truly ready inside to fly... you will succeed... Right now, you could fly and even enjoy it...

You can achieve even more... you can become an overachiever... because you can feel this new strength every day, even when you don't need to fly... every single day, because courage and inner strength show up every day in your posture, in every interaction with others... You move confidently through your daily life... Situations that once may have made you uncomfortable become much easier for you, because inner strength and courage don't just show up when you're flying... In your everyday life, you'll notice this change... and in the coming days, you'll be surprised and pleased at how strong and confident you feel... and how strong and confident others perceive you to be...

Now, focus on the strength within you and at the same time imagine that you are at an airport watching planes take off... and you feel completely at ease because it's so simple... Imagine that you are sitting in the plane, and it's taking off with you and climbing into the sky... and you feel completely comfortable... maybe you think this is only happening here in trance... only here in fantasy... but remember... It's your thoughts that can control your feelings... and your thought... I can and will fly whenever and wherever I want... now leads to calmness, and this exact thought will also lead to calmness when you're flying in the waking state... because even then it is your thoughts that keep you calm... especially this one new thought... I can and will fly whenever and wherever I want...

You've made a decision... You've mastered the fear because your decision is good and constructive... You focus on the thought... I can and will fly whenever and wherever I want... and this thought keeps you calm and will continue to calm you... This thought relaxes your body... and it helps you to be stronger even in your daily life... Your thought helps you to stay calm long before you fly... and your thought helps you stay calm just before flying and even fly with ease... perhaps even with joy, who knows... I can and will fly whenever and wherever I want...

Hypnosis 2

You want to overcome the fear of flying, to be able to fly freely and calmly... naturally and easily... To do this, you've decided to look deep within yourself and sort out everything that has been left unresolved... Today, you're embarking on a journey to yourself... Your journey leads you to yourself... Every thought you think today, every feeling you experience today, brings you closer to yourself... This path is the path of change and renewal... It leads into and through the land of your dreams... There, everything is possible and you can achieve anything, truly anything...

Your journey can begin now... Turn your gaze inward... as if you want to look deep inside yourself, and that's exactly what it's about because the land of dreams lies deep within you... It's always been there, so you don't need to create it... Just turn your gaze inward and focus only on yourself... only on your feelings and let this beautiful land unfold in images... You will find the images of the dreamland within you, I'm sure... with every breath, you come closer to this place in your deep imagination, and you can explore it... Now...

You feel fear when you imagine entering an airplane, and even more fear when you think about flying in it... You avoid flying because of this, but you have the desire to overcome this fear... to fly with a good feeling... The land of dreams is a magical place... Every person can travel to this land... Every person even has their own, very personal dreamland... including you... It is the land of your feelings, and that means you can find your fear of flying there, but not just find it, you can dissolve it as well... Everything can change in the land of dreams if you want it to... that's why you're here... because you want to dissolve the fear... You are ready to process and overcome the fear of flying and its causes in and through the land of dreams and to be free...

You look around and you see a garden... This is the Garden of Time... The gate is wide open, and you enter the garden... There are many areas with blooming plants and well-tended beds... as if a gardener is here every day, keeping everything clean and caring for the plants... But there are also beds lying fallow... and others with dried-up or wilted plants... Some things the gardener may not always tend to enough... other things may no longer be needed or should be removed... Everything has its own special meaning in the Garden of Time... and today, you are here to learn the colors of the dreamland...

The first thing you come to is a pile of gray stones... Gray is the burdensome and heavy in our lives... Humiliations and injuries, losses and failures... Gray also represents what led to your fear of flying... Gray is also everything that has caused or contributed to your fear of flying not yet being overcome and released... Even if there is much gray in your life or was... There was and is also something else... life can also be colorful and bright... But sometimes we no longer see that when we only look at our gray pile of stones... But you're taking a new and different path here, and that's why you look forward and keep moving... towards the colors of the dreamland...

You come to a cherry tree in bloom, its white blossoms shining so brightly that you've already forgotten the gray stones... White is indeed the color of cleansing in the land of dreams... Whenever you encounter it, you recognize that an inner cleansing is taking place... that the gray shadows of the past are fading... that the gray stones that once blocked your way or made you stumble are crumbling to dust because you have processed the painful and bad events of your life... Then it becomes bright and clear within you... Once the fear of flying has been eradicated, your mood brightens as well... that's also what the color white stands for...

You move on through the garden and come to a tree already bearing ripe, red cherries... Strange, you think... Blossoms on one tree and ripe fruits on another... But isn't it like that in our lives... Some things are just emerging... others are growing and flourishing, and still, others are already ripe, just like the time is now ripe for letting go of the fear of flying... and still, others are fading away... withering or drying up in the garden because you no longer need them... or no longer want them... Red is the color of love, and everything red here reminds you of self-love... It is the key to every inner liberation... to every development... to achieving your goals...

You continue through this special Garden of Time, thinking about letting go... You need to and can let go of the fear of flying and with it your feelings of guilt because you often thought that something was wrong with you or that it was your fault, but you didn't choose to have this fear... For inner letting go, you now discover a bed of light blue forget-me-nots... Light blue is the color of overcoming and letting go... Letting go of the fear of flying and also the feeling of shame... This is best achieved when you can accept your own life story with all the events you have experienced... There is only this one life story in your life, you don't have another... you cannot separate from it anyway... If you accept it, then you can let go of many things... Let go of fear and insecurity... Let go of the fear of flying...

You move on and come to a beautiful sunflower... It shines wonderfully golden yellow, so strong and vibrant... The color golden yellow is the color of learning, recognition, and understanding in the land of dreams... That's what it's about... It's not important to know everything or to do everything perfectly... We wish for that, but no one can achieve it... Much more important is to learn... to process what happens to us and to draw our conclusions from it... and to build experience... The color golden yellow in the land of dreams always reminds you of that... wherever and whenever you encounter it...

You've surely often imagined how wonderful it will be once the fear of flying has completely dissolved and you can actually fly with a good feeling... and for that, there is a special tree in the Garden of Time... It bears silver blossoms... You now stand under this tree that cannot exist in your waking life, for silver blossoms only exist here... in the land of dreams, because here there is always, always hope and optimism, and that is the meaning of the color silver... But even in your waking life, there is always hope and optimism... there is always the prospect of a better next day... But we don't always see it that way in our waking life... that's why we don't see the silver tree there either... But you are in the land of dreams and here you recognize the chance for a constructive and therefore silver future without the fear of flying...

Finally, you come to a golden spring... It seems as though pure gold is flowing from this spring, and that is something very special... because gold is the most valuable color in the land of dreams... Gold is the color of life... the color of creation, if you believe in God or a creator... Everything golden in the land of dreams helps you to achieve your goals and to walk your personal path... your golden power helps you at all times... especially when it comes to letting go of the fear of flying...

Then you close your eyes and dream a beautiful dream of how free you will be once the fear of flying is gone forever... The land of dreams helps you with this... because the land of dreams is deep inside you... It has always been there... I'm just telling you about it..

Hypnosis 3

Anchor Technique (Body Anchor, Post-Hypnotic)

As an anchor (or trigger), we refer to a stimulus that is supposed to evoke a specific feeling or awaken a particular thought. It is a signal that the client perceives and then triggers an inner process. The established anchor then replaces the suggestion. In everyday life, a client can use an anchor to trigger or create a desired state, even without being in a trance state. Numerous stimuli can be used as anchors/triggers. I work with the following possibilities, which I also use in the series "Ten Hypnoses": Body anchors (closing the hand, pressing the ball of the thumb...), visual anchors (symbols, word cards...), auditory anchors (signal sounds like mobile phone rings, melodies...), olfactory anchors (scented oils...), tactile anchors (worry stones, talismans...). Additionally, I differentiate between peri-hypnotic and post-hypnotic anchors. Peri-hypnotic anchors are those that are primarily used during hypnosis, where the therapist establishes the anchor and then repeatedly triggers it as a supplement to the suggestions and visualizations.

Post-hypnotic anchors are primarily set up for the time after the session, so the client can help themselves with them.

You have realized that it is possible to overcome the fear of flying... You have realized that it can actually be done, and more than that... You have decided that you want to go down this path... You want to overcome the fear... and there are two ways to do this... You can let go of the fear now... you can use the trance to prescribe yourself a new thought... a thought against fear, which can only be a thought of relaxation, because only one of the two is possible... fear or relaxation... relaxation or fear... and relaxation makes fear impossible... So, today, you can experience relaxation here and counteract any possible fear... prevent any possible fear...

The second option is this... You can learn in the trance to achieve relaxation very quickly, faster than is normally possible in the waking state... because that way, you can experience relaxation even when fear might arise... when it hints at itself, you can counteract it with relaxation... and we'll do both... we'll use the trance for relaxation today and new thoughts of liberation... and we'll use an anchor so that you can always help yourself in everyday life, freeing yourself from thoughts of fear... not letting them arise in the first place... an anchor is a tool... a tool that acts like a switch... a switch against fear... we just need to set it up, and it's easier than you think... We'll do it together... and we'll use anchors that you always carry with you... your hands... You can never forget them... So, you don't have to think about it... no need to carry an object with you... just being present is enough... and maybe you're already wondering how it works, how your hands become the fear-off switch... So, let's go... Experience it today... We'll begin...

You must be calm and free of fear... Now, it's easy... at this moment, you are well relaxed, in a very pleasant trance, and you are following my voice in a relaxed and easy manner, which is guiding and leading you... and if you think you should be even more relaxed, then make yourself as comfortable as possible on the surface that supports your body... and delve deeper into your thoughts, which slowly fade into nothingness... Fear is now far away... You can hear the word fear and even think about fears... remember fear, but stay relaxed... Fear is like a heading over past experiences... now, there is only calmness within you... Stay calm... only my voice guides you... My voice leads you into a comfortable relaxation... and that's what matters... deep calmness... You sink deeper and deeper into the beautiful state of inner calm... you sink very deep into the state of inner calm... well done... very good... You're doing excellently... You're becoming calmer and calmer... and you're focusing all your attention and care on the feeling of relaxation... just like that... exactly like that...

Fear is just a memory that now flows into your hands... now close your hands tightly and imagine that you become even calmer inside when you open your hands again, because your arms relax in the process, and you continue to relax... Keep your hands closed... [Make sure the client actively follows the prompt; if necessary, prompt again. It's not about ideomotor closing of the hand, but an active action.] ...Now open your hands, let go, and feel the relaxation in your arms... Your arms relax, and you become calmer... once more... Close your hands tightly... and let go again to feel the relaxation... Feel the relaxation... Your arms relax, and you become calmer... Do it once more so your body gets used to this rhythm... Close your hands tightly...

and let go again to feel the relaxation... Feel the relaxation... Your arms relax, and you become calmer... The switch works... It works now and whenever you need your fear-off switch... Now, closing and opening your hands puts you into a deeper state of calm, deeper than before... This happens always and everywhere when you use your fear-off switch... Close and open your hands, and the fear disappears... Close and open your hands, and you are relaxed and calm...

Whenever you need it, you can use your fear-off switch, every day... You close and open your hands until the fear disappears... This works very quickly because you can train this switch... even without fear... You can trigger it a few times every day... Just remember that consciously closing and opening your hands turns off the fear, and use this fear-off switch several times... this way, you train the switch, and it gets better and faster every day, better and faster every day... and if you need it before flying or on the plane, it works perfectly for you... Closing and opening your hands drives away any fear... Closing and opening your hands is like throwing away the fear... throwing away the useless fear... Throw away the fear every day... Throw away the fear when you're waiting for your flight... Throw away the fear when you're on the plane... during takeoff, and whenever you think it helps... because it helps you today and every day...

Hypnosis 4

Now, move into relaxation... It's about letting go of all thoughts now, and maybe you're wondering how to do that most easily... Thoughts keep coming back... So imagine that your thoughts come and go... and that every thought that comes flies away... like each thought is a silk scarf that is simply caught by the wind and flies through the air... Then it would be almost impossible to hold on to a thought... Imagine that each thought has a color... then the next thought is green, and a green silk scarf is caught by the wind and flies away... The next thought might be yellow and is also caught by the wind like a fluttering silk scarf and rises into the air... Just imagine lots of yellow thoughts, maybe ten or a hundred silk scarves fluttering through the air... and more are added... whenever a thought could arise, a colored silk scarf of the thought appears and flutters away in the wind... in blue... or red... or purple... in all imaginable colors... The more vividly you can imagine the fluttering scarves in the wind, the faster your thoughts move on and leave you calm... calm and open to new thoughts... open to new and good thoughts that can help you...

Imagine a display board like at an airport... but the display board is completely empty... nothing is displayed there... maybe you remember the old display boards from the past and that typical sound when the letters and numbers would turn, showing a new display... or you only know the new, digital version... where flight times and information appear like on a computer screen, completely silently... Imagine you are standing in front of such a display board within yourself... But here, no flights are being announced... here, more important information about your feelings is being announced... and at this moment, the board changes and shows you a very important message, just for you... It says in bold letters...

Inner calm carries me above the clouds, Inner calm guides me on the way.

... [Read the affirmation slowly and slightly louder than the previous text to emphasize it. Then pause for about 30 seconds before continuing to read.] ...

Now, take a deep breath in... and slowly and fully exhale... once more... [Now, in the client's breathing rhythm]... deep breath in... and slowly and fully exhale... This way, this valuable information can sink in deeper... this way, the words on the display board can become your own words... this way, this exact attitude can become a deep truth within you, and you can truly build this feeling... you can feel the calm now within you... calm that is now possible... calm that is now very simple... calm that is now particularly comfortable... This is how this new connection is created within you... this is how your body learns to connect this calmness with the flight... because everything that is possible in trance is also possible in the waking state... everything that succeeds in the imagination also succeeds in real action... So now enjoy this exact feeling of calmness and imagine that it will soon accompany you when flying... that soon what you see on the display board... what you heard in my words, will become true... a very deep and strong truth within you...

Repetition and Integration of the Affirmation

Deep within your inner core, at the place of your moods and feelings, these words work, which you can read once more on the display board to make them even stronger...

Inner calm carries me above the clouds, Inner calm guides me on the way.

... Now, take a deep breath in and out... let your breath flow calmly, and allow yourself to do nothing... You may relax and rest and think about whatever you want... Everything important has already been done... everything is already taken care of...

Very well... it is time... Everything within you has already adjusted to calmness while flying, and everything will now be different from before... easier... and you can still strengthen your new belief, that's very simple... Just close your eyes for a moment in a quiet moment in the morning and evening and repeat your inner attitude, speak it out loud... Inner calm carries me above the clouds, Inner calm guides me on the way... then this attitude will become more and more stable, and it will be impossible not to feel calm while waiting for the flight... and it will be impossible not to feel calm while flying...

Hypnosis 5

... You have often wondered why you feel guilty when you're afraid, especially when it comes to your fear of flying... We usually feel guilty when we've done something wrong, something we've caused, but you haven't... You didn't choose to have a fear of flying... When you think about your conscience, you quickly realize that you've often struggled with it... even when it wasn't about you and your decisions or actions...

Somehow, you always thought you should do as much good as possible... help as many people as possible and prevent harm from coming to them... a noble thought, but you even took on the guilt for others... This allowed them to feel relieved and innocent... You carry their feelings of guilt to this day, but that should come to an end... because these feelings of guilt were never your own feelings, never your true emotions...

You stand on a high plateau in the land of dreams and look over the land... You look towards the horizon, which seems incredibly far away... But everything is somehow close in the land of dreams, no matter how far away it may seem... When your gaze and therefore a thought go towards the horizon, it's as if you were already there... At the horizon, the future begins in the land of dreams... and since you can be there with just a thought, your future begins right now... in this very moment... or... with the next blink of an eye... and everything is possible there... truly everything...

... Then you move forward because you have the need and the urge to accomplish something... and suddenly you find yourself in front of a wall... It's suddenly there, a gray wall so high that you cannot see over it... This wall stretches across the land of dreams, seeming to divide it into two parts... Gray is the color of pain and suffering in the land of dreams, but also of unresolved conflicts and problems... These often stand like an inner wall before us, towering up... limiting what we can see and understand... You carry many feelings of guilt within you that actually don't belong to you... and these feelings of guilt slow you down and limit you because you believe that you don't deserve happiness or success... Certainly, we all make mistakes and can also bear guilt... But much of what you blame yourself for is not your failure or your doing... You also feel guilty for not being able to save everyone and everything... for not being able to fix everything that life has bent out of shape... These old feelings of guilt should no longer limit you... It is time to finally overcome this supposed guilt... You turn around and suddenly there is also a wall a few steps behind you... You look to the right and left and find yourself enclosed by walls on every side... It is as if you are suddenly enclosed in a gray structure... These are the walls of a guilty conscience and feelings of guilt that trap you here... You would like to break through them...

... Then you remember things that once broke in your life... Maybe there were objects that fell, like plates or cups... Maybe as a child, you broke a vase or another object... perhaps even on purpose, out of anger or revenge... or it was simply carelessness or bad luck... Perhaps you were punished for it, or someone scolded you... You felt guilty... Maybe you managed to hide it and avoided punishment, but you still felt guilty... maybe even to this day, who knows... So many things can break... even inside you... and somehow, you repeatedly believe that you did something wrong or still try to hide that something happened... hiding that you feel bad... perhaps you even tried to hide your fear of flying because you feel guilty about that too... didn't want to be a burden to others... It's time to let go of this guilt today... You don't have to hide anything anymore... Today, you finally let go... You think back... As a child, you often felt lonely and helpless... You needed help as a child... someone to tell you that you are good and lovable... Every child needs that, and every adult needs that too... No one is enough for themselves... We all need people who accept us as we are... But you didn't experience it that way... you simply didn't feel it that way... So, a sad and searching part of you has remained that still believes it was your fault for being alone and lonely... This part of you still hopes that one day someone will be there to catch you and hold you... This someone is here now, you are this someone... You give yourself the support and love that was once missing...

... You wonder what you can do to get rid of these old feelings of guilt that were never your own... How can you break through the guilty conscience... Can you even break it? ... Yes, you can... and you are allowed to, because most of that guilty conscience and those feelings of guilt you took on only for others, to relieve them... to do them a favor, but you don't want that anymore... You want to be free, and that's what you're taking care of today... you're taking care of it now... And suddenly, you have a thick, heavy hammer in your hand... It has a long handle and is so big and powerful that you could knock down walls with it... and that's exactly what it's about... breaking down the wall of guilty conscience and feelings of guilt... This wall is also the wall of fear, the wall of your fear of flying because the two are closely connected... feelings of guilt and fear... If you break down one, the other collapses as well... If you break down the wall of guilt and guilty conscience, the fear falls with it... So, you take the hammer and swing it high... and with all your strength, you strike it against the wall... with all your will for freedom and with all your pent-up anger and inner pain... And then a crack runs through the wall in front of you and simultaneously through all the walls that stand like barriers around you... You wait for a moment, and with a thunderous crash, the entire walls collapse... The guilty conscience has collapsed... The fear of flying has shattered with it... You feel safe and strong again... and with a secure and confident feeling, you move forward, towards the horizon... free of fear and full of confidence, especially when flying... So you move forward... step by step...

Hypnosis 6

Today is the day you want to change your fear of flying... You want to overcome the fear... you want to let it go... Fear is a powerful and forceful energy, so let's change this power... then it can help you... Imagine you could transform fear into courage... simply turn the fear of flying into flying courage... Maybe you're wondering how that can be done... how such a thing can work best... It is possible... it can actually be that simple... We transform your fear of flying into flying courage, and for that, you'll meet a special helper today... or a helper, who knows... You align yourself with all your will and all your strength to work with this helper to transform fear into courage... and thus actually conquer the fear...

Deep inside you, there is a place of silence... The place of silence is a space for encounters... a space for an encounter with yourself... When we meet ourselves at the place of silence, it is different from looking into a mirror, because in a mirror we only see what we want to see... or just what we are used to seeing... But at the place of silence, we meet a special part of ourselves... a part of our personality that can help us solve a problem or get out of a difficult situation more quickly... It is an inner helper that we can meet there, and this inner helper has many faces... Often, it appears as figures and people we once knew who helped us in our lives... You now sink deeper and deeper into your feelings... immerse yourself in yourself, and come closer to the place of silence... It becomes increasingly silent within, and my voice guides you there, to the place of silence... You arrive there, it is a place in your imagination where two airplane seats stand side by side, just like in an airplane...

And now, a person comes to you whom you know from your life... a person who once helped you the most to cope with a difficult situation in your life... or to overcome a hard phase, a time of threat or loss... Maybe it's someone who still helps you today... or it's someone who only helped you once, but so significantly that this is the best helper for the day... Maybe you're also meeting someone who is no longer alive, but at the place of silence, any person can be there as an inner helper... Your inner helper arrives and stands by you as your flight companion... The person who is with you sits down in the seat next to you...

You think about the fear... You are most afraid of flying, but there were other fears in your life too... Fears you've overcome... perhaps this helper, who is with you, even helped you with that... or you didn't realize that it was precisely this helper who had given you support... Sometimes we learn from people without knowing it, or we learn entirely different things than we thought... The person with you tells you that they too have fears about certain events... and that fear is easier to change when there is a helper... and you have a helper... Your helper or companion sits beside you as your flight attendant... first in your imagination and then during the actual flight in your waking state... Your helper has two items with them... a suitcase and a logbook... a logbook with important information about the flight... You think about the fear, about what makes you afraid of flying... maybe you've already found some answers to that... and have an idea of why flying is associated with so much fear... or perhaps you can't quite explain it... and maybe there's a bit of both... reasons for the fear that you know well and some question marks... because the fear seems excessive to you, and you want to overcome it... turn it into courage... Sometimes new insights help... Your flight companion, this inner helper, is with you today because you can learn something special from this person within you, something you don't yet know... Your flight companion opens the logbook... It looks like a thick notebook... The flight companion hands you the book, and in a special way, it's not just the person you think of, but it's a part of yourself that meets you here in this exact form... You look into the book... It says... I'm afraid of flying because that's how you felt before... Then you turn the page, and there is an answer, there is written why it was so... maybe a word or a picture that you can see... Let whatever you perceive be there and just accept it... even if it's something you wouldn't associate with the fear, because our feelings sometimes take strange paths... You think about what the book tells you... and then you close it because whatever it is that's written there, it belongs to the past and should stay there... [Pause for about ten seconds, then continue reading]... Then your flight companion opens the suitcase, and you place the logbook inside, the book of your former fear... because what you once experienced may be a memory and should be an experience, but you no longer need the fear... because the fear has nothing to do with flying...

Your inner helper gets up and takes the closed suitcase away because you don't need it now... when you disembark, you can take the suitcase back and deal with the fear if you want... but you don't need it during the flight... and when you're flying in your waking life, your inner helper will again lock the fear in a suitcase that you hand over and only pick up after the flight... During the flight, your helper accompanies you...

Hypnosis 7

The following hypnosis works with the connection between emotion and body. Since all feelings, as well as thoughts, are reflected in physical reactions—sometimes clearly, often subtly—by focusing on body sensations and attentively addressing the body's signals, the solution to the problem can be worked on. The client should be able to physically feel their deep-seated emotions and thus react more quickly to signs of emotional change. Suggestive techniques help to influence bodily sensations to also change emotions, as not only do feelings create physical reactions, but targeted bodily action also affects feelings. For example, joy creates a smile, and in reverse, intentionally smiling also tends to lift the mood.

Important: Do this hypnosis preferably in a sitting position. Offer the client an armchair or chair with a high backrest so that they can lean both their shoulders and head while sitting. This increases the effectiveness of the approach chosen here.

Today, you want to achieve something special, and the special things are possible in a nice trance... and you are already in a trance... You want to fly without fear... but there is more... Flying without fear is wonderful and liberating... but flying with a feeling of confidence and strength is even better... That will be your goal today because it is possible... Flying with a really good feeling... You've dreamed of this for a long time... Today, this dream will come true... flying with a secure and strong feeling will become your reality, and perhaps you are already curious about how that will be achieved...

Bodily sensations are closely connected to inner feelings, our moods, and emotions... Uncertainty and fear affect posture, just as confidence and assurance do... Confidence leads to a stable posture... with a raised head and straight shoulders... If you imagine sitting in an airplane now and feeling very secure... secure and strong, then you would sit upright... with your shoulders leaning against the backrest, so you can breathe freely and feel free... our body adapts to our feelings, our feelings also adapt to the body... Thoughts of strength and power bring your body into an upright and stable sitting position, and then fear is no longer possible...

Fear must go... So, today you focus on a thought of strength, on a thought of your inner strength... on the thought that you are truly strong, really strong and free from fear... and your body helps you with that... It's remarkable how quickly your posture has already adjusted, right now, in this moment... maybe you noticed it, or maybe you didn't think about it at all, and it just happened... Your body has aligned with strength... your shoulders have moved into a straight and strong position... Your body is preparing everything for you to sit upright and with straight shoulders in the airplane and feel comfortable... That's really possible because you imagine it that way now, and your body follows your imagination... because now, in the trance, you visualize it exactly like this, creating an inner image... because your body always follows your thoughts, and your feelings follow your body... First, there is a thought of confidence and strength, and then your body takes on this posture of confidence and strength... just like now, sometimes unnoticed and all the more effective... and then confidence completely fills you... then strength completely fills you... and fear is impossible... Fear must go... You create an inner image of yourself sitting strong and assured in the airplane, and nothing and no one can shake you... This time has now come, because already now your body is preparing to reduce fear and build strength and become stronger and stronger... Your entire being is strong, much stronger than before... You can and will fly in an airplane and remain calm because you sit upright and stable in your seat... upright and stable, because in this upright posture, you cannot experience fear... If you now consciously feel into your body, you can clearly perceive that it has changed... that your body has changed its posture... adopted a posture of strength... You can perceive it now... You can perceive it very clearly... This is your strength... This is your inner strength... So, all your thoughts align with being very strong and flying as a matter of course... Today, you can feel in your bodily sensation that you already have the power and strength for this... and you will always have it... you will always be able to use your strength whenever you need it... Now is the time to let go of the fear... You know that your fear is now just a memory... a memory of a long-gone time... In this new strong posture, you now free yourself from old thought patterns and habits that you no longer need... You simply lay the fear aside... You simply lay the fear aside by adopting an upright and strong posture... with your shoulders leaning against the backrest... Now feel your shoulders even more clearly... Lean your shoulders against the backrest of your chair and feel the contact because this way you can feel clearly that you are sitting upright... Now imagine you are in an airplane and stay calm... It is impossible not to remain calm and strong because this is a strong posture... So now keep contact with the backrest, and you will remain in this strong position... Now feel intensely into your body... perceive the sensation of your body... Feel the power of your upper body and also your legs... and search for the fear... it's only there as a memory, as a heading or as a note... but you cannot feel afraid now, that's not possible... A strong posture of the body makes fear impossible, prevents any fear...

What you experience now applies every day because your body helps you always and everywhere just like today... Whenever you want to let go of fear or make sure it doesn't even arise, sit down and straighten your body... Lean your shoulders against something so that you can feel that they are truly straight and upright, and immediately the fear disappears... immediately you feel confident and strong... And when you're on an airplane and sit down in your seat, sit upright, lean your shoulders and head against the backrest of the seat, and immediately you feel confident and strong... strong enough for any flight... strong enough...

Hypnosis 8

Ideomotor Techniques

Ideomotor response refers to the phenomenon where our body moves in response to our feelings and thoughts. In everyday life, this response shows up as posture, muscle tension, and movement patterns, which naturally change with mood and thoughts. In trance, ideomotor signals can be used to gain information that the client may not actively communicate. For example, the subconscious can answer questions with a pre-arranged finger signal. Of course, ideomotor responses can also be used suggestively, for example, with arm levitations and catalepsies. An ideomotor approach strengthens trust in hypnosis and in the ability to change, thus promoting therapy.

Important: The following approach is a kind of demonstration in trance. The client should experience that with a simple trick, they become unable to open their hand, and in trance and in the subsequent discussion, they should realize that mental beliefs can maintain problems but can also change them. If you are worried that the hypnosis might not succeed, try it out with a colleague or a friend. Suggestively ensuring that the client's hand can no longer be opened does not require any stage hypnosis skills. It's really simple and almost always works. The "aha" effect is usually quite clear, and belief in hypnosis is strengthened. Further applications in follow-up sessions work accordingly faster and more effectively. Please consider the text as a guide. You must ensure that the fist is closed; if necessary, add more suggestions until the fist is tightly closed. But don't worry – this will rarely be necessary.

Fear of flying has occupied you for a long time... but more than that, you've been occupied with the attempt to end it... Sometimes it's not so easy to let go of a fear, but sometimes it becomes suddenly very easy when we understand the principle of fear... because every fear follows a basic principle... let's just call it the fear pattern... as soon as you understand the fear pattern and recognize that it's nothing more than a stubborn thought, it can also be resolved... because until now, you believed that fear was not influenceable... or only very difficult to influence... this thought is understandable, but it blocks your liberation...

Today, I want to show you that a strong inner conviction makes the impossible possible... A strong conviction can create or maintain fear... but a strong conviction can also end fear immediately...

Focus on your right hand and imagine you have a very valuable object in your hand... an object you absolutely want to hold onto... You want to hold onto it, and that's why your hand closes into a fist... your right hand closes by itself into a fist... the fingers are drawn to the palm as if both were magnetic... your fingers close into a fist, and the fist becomes tighter and tighter... Imagine a valuable object in your hand, perhaps a valuable coin... and your fist closes tighter and tighter... tighter and tighter, your fist closes... tighter and tighter... Your fist becomes tighter and nothing and no one can open it... Your fist closes tighter and tighter... Imagine it, and it will happen... Your fingers close tighter and tighter into a fist... tighter and tighter... tighter and tighter... If someone tried to open your fist, it would close even tighter... I'm going to try to open your fist now, and as soon as I touch it, it will close very tightly...

[Touch the client's closed hand and try to open it. Make sure you clearly feel the resistance. The fist is ideomotorically closed when you touch it. Please do not overdo it, it's not about a test of strength, and you should not succeed in opening the client's hand. If you do succeed or the hand gives way, deepen the trance and strongly suggest the closing of the fist. But don't worry – this will hardly ever be necessary.]

... Your fist is tightly closed... and even if you tried to open it, it would close even tighter... as soon as you try to open your fist, it closes tighter... [Now, timing is important]... Try to open your hand now... [Observe the hand. As soon as you see the client trying to open the hand, "fire" the following suggestion]... and it closes tighter, your fist remains closed... Try it again... Try to open your hand... [Please wait. Usually, the hand cannot be opened anymore, without further suggestion. If that's the case, leave it at that. If there is a slight opening of the fingers, "fire" another suggestion to close]... And why is that? ... because you believe it, because I suggested it to you, and because you tell yourself that it's true... Just as you believe in the closed hand that you cannot open, you also believe in the fear... you still do...

Now imagine something completely different... Imagine your hand is made of rubber and very flexible... a very soft and flexible hand... Imagine your hand is in complete relaxation... your hand relaxes and is loose... calm and loose, as soft and flexible as rubber... Your fingers become very soft and weak... very, very weak your fingers become now and let it happen... Let your fingers become very flexible and soft... and move them a little... It works, you can move them very easily... Your fingers become soft and pliable... very flexible... You can move your fingers again... and open your hand... Open your hand, because you can... And why is that? ... because you believe it... because you know it's possible... because you are sure you can move your fingers... You can open your hand, you can let go of the fear... it all depends on your conviction... only on your belief... Letting go of fear is like opening your hand... very simple... really very simple...

Discuss the process with the client. Explain again that the fear of flying is like a closed fist with the simultaneous belief that letting go is impossible. But with a change of thought, the attitude towards fear changes. This hypnosis can be very well combined with the anchor technique from Main Part 3. That part also deals with opening and closing the hand, but as a symbolic action that becomes an anchor. My classic and tip for you in the treatment of fear of flying: one session with the ideomotor technique presented here, and a week later, a session with the anchor technique (Part 3). Works great!

Hypnosis 9

You want to achieve something... You want to be free from fear and courageous when flying... You want to be able to board an airplane and fly with ease and calmness... That's why you're here today... that's why you're taking action, taking an important step today... It's about a change within you... a change that can be achieved with a single, decisive step when the right moment has come... and maybe today is that moment... in this very moment, it could already be here, or in a few moments...

Perhaps you've often thought there must be a trick to free yourself from the fear of flying... or a good technique... and that's exactly what there is... a trick that is the best technique... You can lose the fear in one step and replace it with ease... simply flying with ease... totally relaxed and light... For this, you need a very good and helpful thought, a formulation of your goal, and at the same time a harmonization of your body, because a harmonious bodily sensation leads to a harmonious mood, and that makes fear impossible... the more you manage to focus on your body and follow a little journey through your body that I guide you on, the faster the fear will fade away and be replaced by ease...

Now, focus on your goal... Fear of flying was in the past... That will be consigned to the past... and so it shall be...

Complete calmness when entering an airplane, and inner lightness when flying

... [When stating the goal formulation, you may also place your palm on the client's solar plexus and then remove it. It's not necessary but helps a lot because the goal formulation is thus "anchored." Of course, you can also incorporate energetic techniques into the hypnosis. Make sure not to repeat the goal.]

Everything now happens deep within you, without any special effort, as long as it succeeds in creating a clear path for the impact of the words heard... Body and mind are directly connected, so it's now particularly important to bring your body into a harmonious state... to eliminate obstacles and blockages in your body... that's very simple... because it can be done with a very specific visualization... So imagine you could breathe into your entire body... not just into your lungs... You know the path of the breath through the nose to the lungs, and you can feel how your lungs fill with air when you inhale... but you can imagine that your breath takes other paths, and the more clearly you can imagine these paths that I show you, the faster your body comes into a harmonious state... and that's what matters... So imagine you could breathe into your arms... When you inhale, the air flows through the nose and trachea to the shoulders and then into the arms... down to the fingertips... and then returns along a harmonious path back to the nose... you find an elegant path for your breath... this creates harmony in your arms... but maybe you have a different visualization... maybe you imagine that the breath gets stuck or diverted somewhere... swirls around... then breathe specifically there, imagine your breath going exactly there, guided by your thoughts and your will... and everything relaxes there, and you find an elegant path for the breath after all... and your arms relax more and more, creating harmony in your arms... and you can also breathe into your upper body and through it... Imagine your breath flowing to the lungs and beyond... into the belly and all the internal organs... like a warm, pleasant stream, your breath flows into your abdomen, enveloping all the organs and flowing back on a harmonious path... maybe through the spine up to the nose... or you find a much more pleasant and harmonious path... and again, if there could be obstacles or blockages anywhere, you know how to eliminate them... Breathe there and experience the harmonization... breathe there and experience the harmony of your body, which now arises... This way, your entire body becomes calmer, more relaxed, and... harmony arises within you... Harmony within you... Go further down to your legs and imagine it again... Your body follows your thoughts and visualizations, so your legs also relax with the same thought... so harmony also arises in your legs with the visualization of breath flowing there... On a harmonious path, the breath flows through the nose... through your upper body... down to the legs... and down to the feet... even down to the toes and back on a harmonious path... and if there could be any obstacles anywhere, you already know how to remove them... So remove all possible obstacles within you and experience the harmony of your body... Experience the harmony of your body now...

Now, only pay attention to your feeling of relaxation and stay in the moment... Everything is done, you don't need to do anything more to let go of the fear... Harmony has already spread and makes fear impossible...

Hypnosis 10

I invite you to a special journey... to a journey through your thoughts and feelings... somewhere in your imagination... But fantasy and reality are only a blink of an eye apart... only a single breath... and every fantasy can become truth if you want it to be so... So you prepare yourself to find a new truth in your life deep in your imagination and creativity... in a land where everything is possible that you can think and dream of... in a land deep within your feelings... in the land of dreams that exists within every person... with just one breath, you reach there... It's time... You enter the land of dreams...

You stand in a meadow... It is a beautiful summer day, and a warm, pleasant breeze is blowing... You look into the distance, your gaze wanders to the horizon... The sky is beautifully blue and clear, without clouds... and birds fly in the sky, carried and driven by the wind... Then you spot a balloon in the meadow, a hot air balloon held to the ground by thick ropes... You walk toward the balloon, and you see a balloonist waving to you, inviting you to take a ride in the balloon... You come closer and closer, and the balloonist comes toward you... He greets you and asks you to get into the balloon because he invites you for a ride... for a gentle flight with the balloon... for a flight over the land of dreams, to look at everything from above in peace... to float above things while being relaxed... In the land of dreams, you cannot have a fear of heights or a fear of flying, not of the balloon flight or the balloon ride, not even of flying with a jet, because the land of dreams is a place of relaxation... a place of beautiful and helpful fantasies... So you climb in, you get into the basket of the balloon, and the balloonist, who will fly with you, gets in too... He will guide you safely... You are in complete safety because in the land of dreams you cannot crash... and even if you were to imagine a crash, nothing could happen to you because you would land on the soft ground of the dreamland... and even the ground of the dreamland is a part of you, like everything else here too... and you never fall deeper in the land of dreams than onto the soft ground of your own soul... so the flight through the air can begin... The lines are released, and the balloon rises slowly into the air... gently and leisurely, the balloon begins to float... It slowly rises into the air... high into the sky, and you look out of the balloon... You look down to the earth... and you are relaxed because it's easy here in the land of dreams... Your flight first goes over a forest... and the forest is always the forest of your own thoughts in the land of dreams... It lies beneath you, and you rise even higher... all fearful thoughts also lie beneath you... You float above them... you are greater than your thoughts of fear... Then you look from up here over the land... You can see everything clearly... you can see meadows and forests... mountains and valleys... rivers and lakes... You can see everything clearly from up here, you can recognize everything... and you can understand everything... Then your flight leads over an ocean, which in the land of dreams is the ocean of feelings...

... Then you notice that there are two gray spheres in the basket of the balloon... You take the first sphere in both hands... it is heavy because it is the sphere of responsibility... Often in life, you have felt responsible, often taken on responsibility... Sometimes responsibility was with you, sometimes it was in other hands, but there was no one who really wanted or could carry it themselves... so you repeatedly took on the responsibility... It took a lot of strength... There was often no time for fear and insecurity, or you acted despite great uncertainty and followed your path... But the sphere of responsibility in this balloon stands primarily for the responsibility you took on that didn't really belong to you or wasn't yours... even for your fear of flying, you are not responsible... it came about, you couldn't choose it... Today, you can let go of this responsibility... You take the gray sphere of responsibility and throw it out of the basket... You watch the sphere as it falls into the ocean and sinks deep down into the water... There it can and will stay... as a memory, as an experience... but it can no longer burden you from there... You no longer want to carry it with you... The balloon becomes lighter and rises higher, and it becomes clear to you that the many responsibilities of your life made up part of your fear... in the overburdening with responsibility over the course of life, over the long time, fear could arise... Fear that had nothing to do with flying but could show itself there... Then you take the second sphere in your hands, grabbing it with both hands... It is the sphere of guilty conscience and feelings of guilt... Often, with all the responsibility, you also felt guilty, thinking you did something wrong... had a guilty conscience when something didn't work out, when you couldn't prevent damage... even when it was impossible for you to prevent it... and upon closer inspection, guilt and conscience are the same feeling... but that wasn't your true feeling, not when you developed a guilty conscience from a responsibility that wasn't yours... So this guilty conscience also contributed to the fear building up over time... and it showed itself where you could do the least – when flying because you can't take responsibility there... you have to leave the responsibility to the pilot... You throw this sphere into the ocean beneath you too... It falls into the water and sinks to the bottom... as a memory, as an experience... and you become lighter, the balloon becomes lighter and rises higher into the sky... it becomes light when flying in the land of dreams...

You feel the lightness and enjoy the flight in the land of dreams... Is this fantasy? ... Or just a fairy tale? ... The land of dreams is real because it is deep inside you... it has always been there... I'm just telling you about it...

All Titles in the Series

Volume 1: Smoking Cessation
Volume 2: Anxiety and Restlessness
Volume 3: Burnout
Volume 4: Reducing Overweight
Volume 5: Coping with the Past
Volume 6: Suicidal Thoughts and Attempts
Volume 7: Psycho-Oncology
Volume 8: Obsessions and Tics
Volume 9: Self-Confidence and Decision-Making
Volume 10: Grief Work
Volume 11: Psychosomatics
Volume 12: Chronic Pain
Volume 13: Depressive Thoughts
Volume 14: Panic Attacks
Volume 15: Domestic Violence, Victim Support
Volume 16: Post-Traumatic Stress
Volume 17: Exam Anxiety and Stage Fright
Volume 18: Anti-Violence Training, Offender Support
Volume 19: Addiction Tendencies
Volume 20: Social Phobia and Fear of Contact
Volume 21: Nail Biting
Volume 22: Self-Awareness and Self-Love
Volume 23: Teeth Grinding and Night Clenching
Volume 24: Feelings of Guilt
Volume 25: Fear in Crowds
Volume 26: Fear of Flying, Aviophobia
Volume 27: Fear in Enclosed Spaces, Claustrophobia
Volume 28: Tinnitus, Ear Noises
Volume 29: Fear of Heights
Volume 30: Neurodermatitis

Volume 31: Finding Inner Balance
Volume 32: Overcoming Loneliness
Volume 33: Fear of Illness, Hypochondria
Volume 34: Anticipatory Anxiety, Fear of Fear
Volume 35: Jealousy in Relationships
Volume 36: Driving Anxiety
Volume 37: New Start after Separation
Volume 38: Fear of Injections
Volume 39: Heart Anxiety Neurosis
Volume 40: Overcoming Resentment and Anger
Volume 41: Resolving Blockages and Positive Thinking
Volume 42: Stress Reduction, Stress Management
Volume 43: Body Relaxation
Volume 44: Deep Relaxation
Volume 45: Fear of the Dark
Volume 46: Falling Asleep and Staying Asleep
Volume 47: Compulsive Buying
Volume 48: Restless Legs Syndrome
Volume 49: Bulimia
Volume 50: Anorexia
Volume 51: Overcoming Nightmares
Volume 52: Imagined Deformity
Volume 53: Overcoming Distrust, Finding Trust
Volume 54: Processing Failures
Volume 55: Humiliation, Emotional Hurt
Volume 56: Distressing Compassion, Vicarious Suffering
Volume 57: Self-Forgiveness
Volume 58: Self-Awareness, Self-Confidence
Volume 59: Saying No
Volume 60: Assertiveness
Volume 61: Setting Boundaries and Self-Assertion
Volume 62: Decision-Making Ability

Volume 63: Success Orientation
Volume 64: Ruminating, Circular Thinking
Volume 65: Accepting Pregnancy
Volume 66: Birth Preparation
Volume 67: Spiritual Opening
Volume 68: Joy of Life and Inner Lightness
Volume 69: Patience and Inner Peace
Volume 70: Fibromyalgia and Rheumatism
Volume 71: Irritable Bowel Syndrome, Crohn's Disease
Volume 72: Fear of Nausea, Emetophobia
Volume 73: Stuttering and Cluttering, Speech Flow Disorders
Volume 74: Concentration and Knowledge Anchoring
Volume 75: Vitality and Spontaneity
Volume 76: Searching for Meaning and Finding Goals
Volume 77: Life Crises, Life Events
Volume 78: Workaholism, Goal Obsession
Volume 79: Helper Syndrome, Helpless Helpers
Volume 80: Medication Abuse
Volume 81: Gambling Addiction
Volume 82: Internet Addiction, Smartphone Addiction
Volume 83: Hoarding Disorder, Compulsive Collecting
Volume 84: Conspiracy Thoughts, Overvalued Ideas
Volume 85: Fear of Operations and Treatments
Volume 86: Fear of Aging
Volume 87: Travel Anxiety
Volume 88: Anxiety When Urinating, Paruresis
Volume 89: Fear of Intimacy and Togetherness
Volume 90: Fear of Blushing
Volume 91: Coming Out in Homosexuality
Volume 92: Charisma Training
Volume 93: Migraines and Chronic Headaches
Volume 94: Overcoming Allergies, Bronchial Asthma

Volume 95: Normalizing Blood Pressure
Volume 96: Compulsive Perfectionism
Volume 97: Sports Hypnosis, Motivation
Volume 98: Sports Hypnosis, Performance Enhancement
Volume 99: Determination and Focus
Volume 100: Encountering the Inner Child
Volume 101: Cravings, Binge Eating
Volume 102: Stimulating Metabolism
Volume 103: Bipolar Mood Swings
Volume 104: Borderline, Identity Crises
Volume 105: Hypomania, Euphoria, Mania
Volume 106: Restlessness, Agitation
Volume 107: Nervous Breakdown
Volume 108: Adjustment Disorders
Volume 109: Self-Alienation, Depersonalization
Volume 110: Ending Self-Pity
Volume 111: Primary Gain of Illness
Volume 112: Secondary Gain of Illness
Volume 113: Bullying, Victim Support
Volume 114: Letting Go of Envy and Jealousy
Volume 115: Fear of Spiders, Arachnophobia
Volume 116: Fear of Dogs or Cats
Volume 117: Fear of Strangers, Xenophobia
Volume 118: Excessive Worries, Generalized Anxiety
Volume 119: Strengthening Sense of Responsibility
Volume 120: Unrequited Love, Heartache
Volume 121: Work-Life Balance
Volume 122: Letting Go of Unattainable Goals
Volume 123: Allowing and Accepting Help
Volume 124: Letting Go of Adult Children
Volume 125: Tourette Syndrome
Volume 126: Life Changes and New Starts

Volume 127: Accepting Life in a Wheelchair
Volume 128: Understanding and Overcoming Homesickness
Volume 129: Understanding and Overcoming Wanderlust
Volume 130: Dizziness, Meniere's Disease
Volume 131: Overcoming Aggression
Volume 132: Cutting and Self-Harm
Volume 133: Hair Pulling, Trichotillomania
Volume 134: Postpartum Depression
Volume 135: For Relatives of Dementia Patients
Volume 136: Self-Harm, Artificial Disorders
Volume 137: Activating Self-Healing Powers
Volume 138: Preventing Depression Relapse
Volume 139: Reactive Psychoses, Follow-Up
Volume 140: Obsessive Thoughts and Impulses
Volume 141: Compulsive Checking
Volume 142: Compulsive Counting, Symmetry Obsession
Volume 143: Compulsive Washing, Cleanliness Obsession
Volume 144: Compulsive Questioning
Volume 145: Dissociative Paralysis
Volume 146: Phantom Pain
Volume 147: Overcoming Complaining
Volume 148: Hay Fever, Pollen Allergy
Volume 149: Sexual Abuse, Victim Support
Volume 150: Standing Strong Against Sexism, #metoo
Volume 151: Binge Eating
Volume 152: Overcoming Thoughts of Revenge
Volume 153: Detachment from the Aggressor, Stockholm Syndrome
Volume 154: Courage to Separate
Volume 155: Chronic Fatigue, Exhaustion
Volume 156: Fear of the Future, Existential Anxiety
Volume 157: Excessive Worry About Children
Volume 158: Fear of Failure

Volume 159: Ending Distrust and Control
Volume 160: Dejection, Dysphoria
Volume 161: Boreout, Chronic Boredom
Volume 162: Bipolar Disorders, Relapse Prevention
Volume 163: Mania, Relapse Prevention
Volume 164: Nihilism, Feelings of Worthlessness
Volume 165: Thumb Sucking
Volume 166: Being Brave
Volume 167: Being Proud
Volume 168: Overcoming Shyness
Volume 169: Being Able to Delegate Responsibility
Volume 170: Being Able to Show Emotions
Volume 171: Letting Go of Guilt, Victim Support
Volume 172: Processing Guilt, Offender Support
Volume 173: Mood Swings, Cyclothymia
Volume 174: Lack of Drive, Vital Sadness
Volume 175: Hearing Voices with Reality Reference
Volume 176: Confident Communication
Volume 177: Standing Up for Oneself
Volume 178: Taking New Paths
Volume 179: Confident Job Application
Volume 180: No Longer Being Taken Advantage Of
Volume 181: End of Submissiveness
Volume 182: Depressive Numbness
Volume 183: Mood Drops, Affective Incontinence
Volume 184: Mood Instability
Volume 185: Somatoform Disorders
Volume 186: Stomach Ulcer, Psychosomatic
Volume 187: Accepting Amputation
Volume 188: Overcoming and Letting Go of Hatred
Volume 189: Ending Accusations
Volume 190: Allowing Tears, Being Able to Cry

Volume 191: Finding and Sorting Repressed Feelings
Volume 192: Somatoform Pain
Volume 193: Living Autonomously
Volume 194: Anhedonia, Joylessness
Volume 195: Persistent Sadness
Volume 196: Obesity, Food Addiction
Volume 197: Parents of Abused Children
Volume 198: Letting Go and Letting Be
Volume 199: Childhood Sexual Abuse
Volume 200: Fear of Loss

www.ingramcontent.com/pod-product-compliance
Lightning Source LLC
Chambersburg PA
CBHW030456220526
45464CB00006B/2555